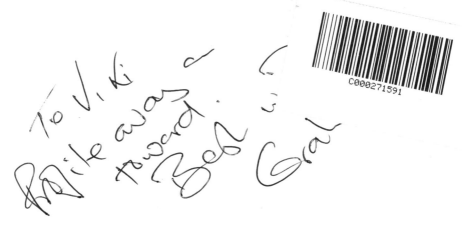

WHO'S BROKEN MY SCALES?

THE WEIGHT MANAGEMENT APPROACH WITH THE FAIRY TALE ENDING

Designed and written by

Jan Russell Dexter, Jayne Hildreth and Graham Dexter

Illustrated by BJ Boulter

ISBN 978-0-9515525-3-7

CONTENTS

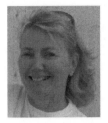 Hi, I'm **Jan Dexter**. I'm a `family woman', a writer and a motivational coach. I enjoy good, fresh food, red wine, and Thornton's chocolate. I also enjoy being active. Weight for me is about feeling good, and being in balance with my mental and physical self. I believe that life is for living to the full, *and* I am passionate about bringing out the best in people.

I use the links between body, language and mind to inspire motivation and create change. I know that in the psychology of sustainable change, we can each be very different - for me, this approach beats the zip zap happy clappy promise that one size fits all, so to speak.

In 2006, I walked the Inca trail. In training, I dropped weight, got fitter and felt terrific. Like many of you, I'm a `Strictly' fan, and would love to do it! However, I can't walk the Inca trail every week, I'm not likely to get onto `Strictly', but I can make walking and dancing ways of keeping fit and feeling fab. Anyone can find their own fancies and styles. I don't think *we* can make you thin, or that everyone wants to be thin. I do believe that *you* can make you the size you want to be – in fact, you're already an expert on that. I might have a few hints on how to use that expertise in the way you want.

So, enjoy this programme, and remember to stop now and then and smell the coffee☺. Look after yourself - because wherever you go, there you'll be.

Warm wishes, *Jan*

I'm **Jayne Hildreth** and I'm a normal woman – whatever that means! Let's say I don't claim I can eat and drink anything and everything whilst miraculously remaining a tiny size 6 (for the record I'm not a size 6 either nor would I choose to be).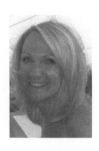

I manage my weight with exercise, balanced eating and very importantly living! I have been told we are only here once so the living part for me is of great significance. I use the gym on a regular basis which works for me. It is an environment which I have learnt to feel comfortable in. I love the feeling of being physically fit and in shape. The gym offers variety which is necessary for me as I have a very low boredom threshold so I need this kind of motivation. In addition, I have a beautiful little Westie who despite having very short legs, loves to walk!

So what qualifies me to co-author this book? Well, aside from walking the walk I have worked with individuals' change needs for the last 15 years, as a therapist and now as a coach. I feel intense irritation when I see negative and judgmental attitudes towards weight loss and in particular the idea that one size and one outcome fits all. In addition I am passionate about facilitating others' changes and relish the opportunity to share my knowledge and expertise to enable you to achieve your desired goals, whatever they may be.

Enjoy this new and exciting journey of doing what works and marvel at the results!

Best wishes, *Jayne*

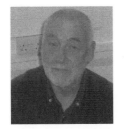I'm **Graham Dexter**, and I'm a bloke. Blokes don't have weight issues, so I was a bit shocked when a medical consultant intimated that I needed to lose about 2 stone. What a cheek. He was saying I was fat! When I checked with the BMI charts, they indicated I was `pre -obese' - what a liberty! Unlike my female colleagues, I don't believe in exercise, the best it gets for me is a walk round the snooker table, and the occasional walk with the dog. I have been known to take a golf buggy and take a few swipes at a ball or two, and then a longer walk to find them, but nothing excessive.

I guess that's why I'm here, to encourage the lazy ones amongst you. I managed to lose my 2 stone effortlessly, and that's what I intend to help you do too – do what you need to easily. I've been a coach, counsellor, therapist and trainer for many years and I think I can share with you a few tricks that will be very helpful. I will also , with your permission, help you relax your way into a state that will make losing weight and getting into the shape you want happen with so little effort you'll wonder why you haven't done it years ago...oh that's right you didn't know me then did you?

See you later, give me a good listening to and relax into your desired shape.

Graham

ACKNOWLEDGEMENTS

We three wrote this book with commitment, professional knowledge, flexibility, a curiousity to find out more, and a willingness to work with each others' strengths and to accept revisions. We've created a book that we believe will support a lot of people to manage their weight a lot more easily.

A number of people deserve acknowledgement. Tony Hildreth helped us to understand our illustration needs. BJ Boulter created the magical illustrations willingly and supportively, and we are so grateful.

For reading transcripts, evaluating titles, and general support, we would like to thank Sara Christensen, Chris Hildreth, Roe and Rodger Holcombe, Debra Jinks, Judi Irving, Adele North, Sue Russell Taylor, Heather Maxfield, Suzy Scroggs.

Many psychologists have influenced us over the years. We would like to acknowledge particularly the work of Prochaska and diClemente, Gerard Egan, Robert Dilts, Richard Bandler, Paul McKenna and of course all the people they learned from as well.

Our clients over the years, and our students, have made us better practitioners, and our practice informs our writing, so thank you to you all.

The book is dedicated to all those people who would love to become comfortable with their weight and become their own host at their particular party of life.

You can, you know.

INTRODUCTION

Welcome to *Who's Broken My Scales*, the weight management approach with the fairy tale ending. This fun and effective programme is designed to assist you to reach the size and shape that realistically suits you and makes you feel great. The programme is based on two major beliefs that the authors have, which prove useful over and over again. One is that your body and mind are so deeply connected that by changing your *mindset*, you will bring long lasting changes for your body. Two, we believe that you can make the necessary switches in your mind once you learn the basic principles outlined in our clear and straightforward programme, in which this short, sharp and tasty book is a key resource.

Before we go any further, a word on how to use the book. Each section can be read on its own to help you to re programme your thinking and approach, so it may be that you only ever read one chapter. Alternatively, you might want to read it all through because it's so effective in helping you to better understand and motivate yourself. If so, you may want to do that either in sequence, or by hopping about to whichever section attracts you most. It's a bit like eating a good meal – you may want one course, or seven; you may want lots of starters; you may want only pudding. It's up to you to find what works. So use this book as a pocket guide to accompany you on your journey of making life in your skin the best it can possibly be. The choice of how to read it fits with the whole message behind this book - **do what works for you**! We are all different.

The sections cover seven easy principles, each associated with simple and familiar stories. ***The Frog Prince*** introduces you to the psychological stages of change. ***Mirror Mirror*** addresses some basic issues about your identity, while ***Aladdin and his Magic Lamp*** helps you to be sure of what changes you want to make. ***The Hare and the Tortoise*** brings to mind the importance of your beliefs, while ***Cinderella*** reminds you of all the capabilities and resources that you have to make those beliefs work for you. In ***Beauty and the Beast*** you learn how to programme and control your behaviours, and in ***Mary, Mary***, you can learn to create the environment you want to support your changes.

Each section has two parts. In the first part, we invite you to read, listen, and consider. In the second half we present structured exercises that you might want to work through. For some people, writing things down can help you to understand them better, and fix things more clearly in your brain. Some people are not so keen to do this. Whatever works for you.

We have an MP3 available which supports this programme. This provides ten easy entrancements which are easy to listen to and effective. One offers you some motivation strengthening through deep relaxation, while the others are more conscious short chunks of reinforcement for each section. So, whether or not you use the book alone or with the MP3, you can choose whatever will be most supportive.

11

You know, sometimes making changes in weight, size or fitness can feel like a real challenge, like climbing a mountain. Well, imagine that it really *is* like a big climb – big climbs can be the most exhilarating and satisfying journeys in the world. Just think about it, and consider how many ways there are to climb a mountain. Imagine you are in a whole group of people doing the same climb – everyone will want to get to different points at different times, some will want to rest and enjoy the view, some will want to get there faster, some will need help, some will give help.

So it is with learning to make changes that last, rather than following fads. Everyone has their own pace and method. In our programme, we are not saying there is only one way, and that's what makes this a little bit different. Your goals are unique to each and every one of you, there is no right or wrong, good or bad - this is all about what *you* want, feeling fabulous and doing what works!

The premise is simple. Assuming that we are talking to people who are not tied up and force fed, the only person that makes you unhappy with your physical self is you. Therefore it's really useful to find out just *how* you do that. We're pretty sure you'll find it's a mix of what you say to yourself, how your words affect your mind, how you respond to situations around you, and what behaviours you then do. You've developed a series of beliefs and habits over the years which have resulted in you having a level of dissatisfaction, or urge to change. This is what has caused you to engage with this programme. Those beliefs and habits have taken a lot of energy and determination to create. The good news is that if you can put that much effort into *mis*management, reprogramming them can only be easier. By understanding your thoughts, language and behaviour, you can channel your energy into treating yourself in a way that pays the dividends you want.

You are your own expert!

Our mission is simple – to help you to change the beliefs and habits which you use and do not like, into beliefs and habits which are more helpful to you. You can learn to reprogramme your mind to shape your body, your way.

A final word. While you read this book, just eat and exercise as you fancy. This is very important – please try this at home!

As you read each section and consider their contents carefully, you are likely to find that you quite easily and naturally start to make small changes. Engage with the stories and the invitations, do the exercises if you want to, and you will discover that those small changes become the foundation of the bigger changes that you might expect over the rest of your life.

Enjoy!

THE FROG PRINCE

UNDERSTANDING THE CYCLE OF CHANGE

How does change happen? Let's start by remembering the story of the Frog Prince who achieved huge transformation from being a small (and bordering on the unattractive) little frog to a

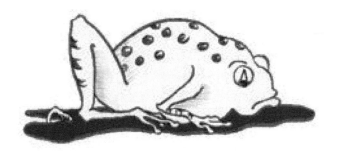

handsome and very eligible prince. We are not for a moment suggesting any of you represent the frog – it's simply that perhaps it is helpful to think about him in a way that highlights the fact that change is always possible when you want it enough ☺.

Consider the change you are choosing to embark on now. How will you make it happen? We feel certain you have all experienced the process of change on many occasions, and are sure you would agree that it doesn't just happen *to* us! To achieve change, we have to *engage* with it and be *active* in it.

Sometimes, part way through the process of change, we might lose track of our progress, lapse into

14

old habits, or think `I've lost track of this', `I'm not getting where I want.' It's like we've fallen off the wagon, because we don't feel sure of where we are, or how to get back on that damned wagon!

Understanding the process of change is really helpful for those moments, and to ensure our sustainable success. There are several theories available that attempt to describe this process. One that is of particular use for weight loss, or shape changing, and which is fully tried and tested, comes from the work of some psychologists called Prochaska and Diclemente. When you become familiar with the ideas based on their theory, you will have a framework, or a map, that you can easily check in with to help you to keep on heading in the right direction.

We believe that when you know where you are, you can then consider where ideally you would prefer to be, and work out how you intend to get there, even if the odd slip off the wagon occurs on the way.

So, let's think back to our frog living in the pond. Top heavy, a little spotty, and accepting his lot. Not even considering any change.

Yet after seeing the Princess, dear old Frog started to think that he really would prefer to be handsome, human and loved. He needed therefore to engage with the change process, and began to think about all the things he might need to consider before swinging into action and wooing the Princess. And we want to invite you to do the same – to engage with your change process.

You can start to check it out by thinking about a time when you have changed something in your life. It may well be around losing weight, as we imagine that most of you reading this book have had some excellent previous experience of this!

How did you do it?

We would encourage you to consider your experience alongside the Frog's story.

Like him, to begin with you probably spent some time not even thinking about change. You might have been quite comfortable in your skin, with your habits, with your size and shape. You might have noticed changes occurring but for whatever reasons remained quite accepting of them. You may have been trying to ignore your size and shape, or it is possible that amongst all the other events and demands in your life, it was something you were not yet paying attention to. You were the Frog in the pond, just enjoying the environment in the great outdoors.

This step in the change process can be described as **pre-contemplation** – a place where you either do not want to change yet, or have not considered it a possibility.

Then, something probably occurred which resulted in you beginning to think about change. Maybe other people were putting pressure on you to alter your behaviour around eating and exercise. It can often be the case that a Doctor or family member attempts to advise a change for the good of your health. (Weight to height ratio, blood pressure, cholesterol, pressure on arthritic joints, for example.) It may be that your stimulus was in reaction to something more internal - a feeling on seeing a photograph, not being able to get into a certain item of clothing, feeling puffed out by climbing the stairs. Maybe you wanted to achieve a challenge that you weren't yet in shape for – just like the Frog.

The impact of such moments or realizations can cause you to leap off the lily pad and view yourself differently, maybe causing strong feelings 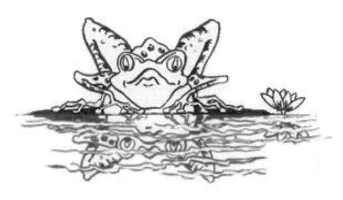 inside. You will doubtless recognise this experience – it can feel uncomfortable, even slightly shocking. The best things about these moments are that you can now be open to the idea that things can be different, even feel good about that, and think 'yes, ok I want to make some changes.'

And then you believe that you really **can** make any changes that you want.

Just as our friend the Frog did when he saw the beautiful princess. He began to think that if *he* could transform himself, then being with her might well be a possibility. He *wanted* to feel different, he began to imagine that he **could** be different, and he wanted to make the Princess sit up and take notice of him. He became motivated. For him, the Princess' beauty (and, obviously, her personality☺) gave him the impetus to change.

This state of being can be described as *contemplation* – now, for whatever reason, you are considering a different future.

Sounding familiar, as you consider changes that you have made in the past?

We don't know about you, but in our experience an urge to act often follows this stage of contemplation. Yet in the process of long term change, it's useful to realize that there are more things to consider before moving to action. It's common for people not to realize this, and many like to dive in and do.

However there is an important stage of **pre-action/ pre planning** in order to make a sustainable difference. Imagine if the Frog, on seeing the beautiful princess, just flew out of the water and flung himself into her arms. The results may well not have been desirable. Rather, you might agree that it was more helpful for him to think a little before taking that leap into action–remember - 'Look before you Leap!'

In your own experience of previous change, what pre planning took place?

❖ What did you need to consider?
❖ What were your actions following this?
❖ And did they achieve sustained change?

Commonly, when people swing into action regarding weight or shape change - `I'm joining the gym', `I'm cutting my calories', `I'm going to walk instead of getting the bus', they begin with great motivation and good intentions.

Over time, they might then experience a *lapse*, a phase where they go back to old behaviours. This might happen during an evening out or on a special occasion for example. It is our view that pre-planning will help to prevent this happening. When you understand more about the cycle of change, you will understand that even if this happens, it is what we *do* about it that matters as much as, or more, than the lapse itself.

Some people go straight into thinking 'well it's ruined now, I've spoilt it completely', and use the lapse as an excuse or reason to abandon the whole change programme, and dive back into the murky waters of dissatisfaction and helplessness. This then leads to full relapse, and abandoning their good work. How many people out there have said such things as `I lost three stone, dropped 2 dress sizes, and now I've put it all back on'?

Others might think 'well, I've spent a day or two in my old habits, now I'll get back on track and balance out what I'm doing so I can get to where I want to be.' When you are armed with the knowledge of how change works, you are more likely to be able to take that approach. You can realize that even with a lapse, you can still take charge of your change process, and choose to think and do differently to your previous attempts in weight management.

This shift in thinking leads to you being able to stay within the change process and achieve your goal. It also enables you to succeed in the final stage of **maintenance**, doing what you need in order to make your changes robust, sustainable, and effective. This is more likely to work if you have done the planning of what 'contingencies' you can have in place if every day hasn't gone as smoothly as you'd hoped.

Does this sound familiar to you?

If you were to think about where you are in this moment in relation to losing weight, what stage are you currently at? The fact that you are reading this book suggests that you are at the very least *contemplating* change, possibly *preparing*, and now considering how to *act.* Our encouragement is to contemplate carefully what you want, prepare thoroughly, think about all the possible actions you can to get to where you want to, and prepare how you might respond if you lapse.

As a final note, remember you are developing your own personal plan so use what fits and works for you.

Oh - and the most really significant point to
remind you of before we finish…

The Frog became a Prince – *and* got his Princess!!

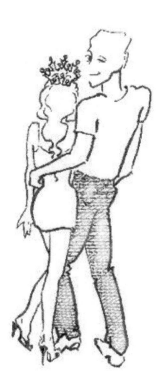

Suggested Exercises

Grab a pen and some paper, as it can be helpful to write things down as you go. Find somewhere comfortable and quiet to sit. Now, allow yourself to think back to a time when you have attempted to lose weight or change something previously. Think about how that journey started for you.

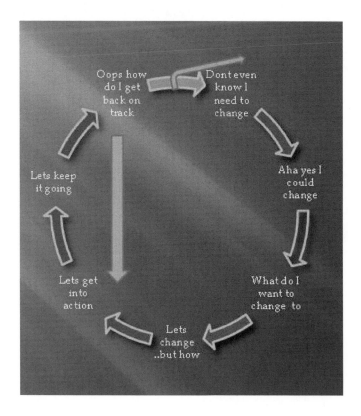

❖ What happened to make you decide you wanted to

embark on this change?

❖ How did you then start to prepare?

❖ What encouraged you?

❖ Once prepared, what kind of things did you do towards achieving your weight loss/change?

❖ What changes did you make? Really give yourself time to think about this in detail, and remember – write your answers down.

❖ Can you remember what kind of thoughts and feelings you had around this time?

❖ What was going well?

❖ What was a little more of a challenge?

❖ How did you manage those challenges? Who or what for example?

❖ To what extent did you manage to consolidate and maintain the change?

If not...

❖ What caused you to lapse/ fall off the wagon?

❖ How did you stay off the wagon?

❖ What did you learn from this?

❖ If you were able to step back in time, what would you do differently?

Now

❖ What has caused you to contemplate more effective weight management now?

❖ What do you need to plan?

❖ What actions need to be in your plans?

❖ With all of your knowledge, what might you pre-plan in case of a lapse?

Write down your three key learnings from doing this exercise:

1.

2.

3.

MIRROR, MIRROR ON THE WALL

A QUESTION OF IDENTITY

Mirror Mirror on the wall, who is the fairest of them all?

How many of you ask yourself that question when you see your own reflection, and how many of you have a mirror that answers `me'?  Our hunch is that not everyone out there is yet as happy with their body image as that Wicked old Queen in the fairy tale of Snow White and the Seven Dwarves. Because it's all a question of how we see ourselves – our `shape identity.'

Our weight and shape often sneak into our whole idea of who we are, don't they, and how we fit into the world. Because issues of weight, and shape run so deeply within us, some people find that in order to control their food, they have to change relationships with significant others. Some are frightened of feeling fabulous. Some people don't find it easy to put themselves first. So, weight and shape become a part of our identity. And we describe others all the time, don't we, by their shape and size - skinny, fat, porky, chubby, thin as a rake, plump, as if the shape defines the person, as if the person *is* the shape.

Sometimes it can feel as if we are permanently on a shape identity parade!

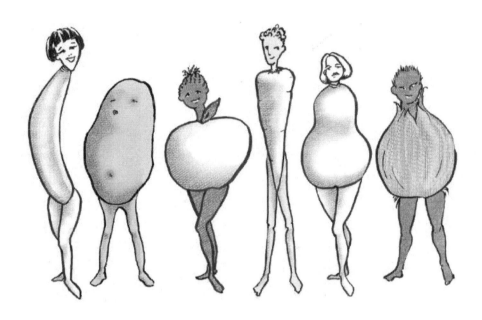

As you are reading this book, chances are you'd like to change your shape identity, or change something in the way you feel about your size and shape. You probably have a great deal of understanding of the story of how/why you have become the shape you are – many of these stories devoid of responsibility and leaning to factors outside ourselves - 'when I started nursing, there were always chocolates on the ward', 'once I had that desk job, I was sitting around a lot', 'I'm on the road a lot, it's hard to take control of my eating', `I always finished the kids' left overs' – we've all done it.

It's also common to unwittingly hide behind a dishonest sense of self, like `I'm not a greedy person', `I'm quite a controlled eater so I don't know why I put weight on', `I have an active job so it's not like I don't exercise', and so on.

Even though we might also be operating secretly on the basis that:

`if a man goes into the kitchen and eats a whole slab of chocolate, and there is no one around to see this happen, does the chocolate still have calories in it?'

It's just that, for whatever reason, we can't *identify* ourselves as a greedy person, or an out of control person. It doesn't sit right, or carries association with guilt, or shame, or naughtiness – whatever it is for you.

And many people have a distorted view of themselves in that mirror. A distorted sense of identity. Some slim people see themselves as fat; some people don't find it easy to accept their own personal beauty.

We can also shape our self-concept by measuring ourselves internally against some global image of `what sort of person' we are. `Oh, I couldn't go to a gym – I'm not that kind of a person', `exercise and me just don't get on', `I use a lift to save my legs', or `I'm not the kind of person who likes to feel physically fit.' We might have images of what physically fit looks like, and if they are too far removed from who we think we are, then we might deny ourselves the enjoyment of being in touch with the physical side of our being.

Yet it's well known that taking part in enjoyable activity can in itself give a sense of accomplishment which feeds your self - concept and therefore your self - esteem. So you might not be the kind of person who joins a gym *(whoever that might be)*, but that's not to say you can't be the kind of person who can become family champ at Wii fit bowls, or someone who could make that walk with the dog a little brisker. You maybe someone who enjoys doing yoga, or someone who questions what it is you're saving your legs for, and instead begins to feel a little fitter and brighter, and experience that as a part of who you are.

So, who are *you* when it comes to your shape identity? How do you think of yourself around size, shape and weight? Can you accept that you are a wonderful person as you are, even if you want to change some bodily aspects?

And can you look at yourself honestly?

Often, people ignore their changing shape for a period of time, either deliberately or just not taking notice – no reason to, feeling fine, doing well at work so replacing clothes on monthly basis not an issue. That's quite a nice place to be, un self – conscious.

Or it can be that you are oblivious to the gasps and stares of people around you, their pitying glances, and their disapproval as you tuck into another vat of ice cream☺

Who are you at this point? You might be the person who doesn't put looks as the highest value, the person who doesn't look in the mirror at all, or the person who *is* the fairest of them all. You may enjoy a greater perspective on life than those who are weight obsessed, or you could be burying your head in the sand.

Then, suddenly, one day, that trusty mirror on the wall let's you know that you are no longer the fairest of them all, and you see yourself, for whatever reason, in a different light.

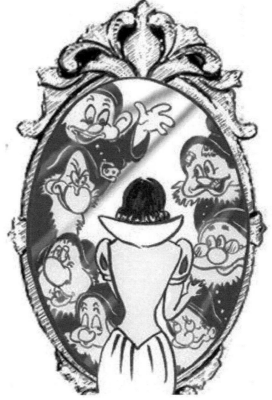

And it's like those seven dwarves have all arrived in your

mirror at once, shouting at you, `who's Greedy, who's Unhealthy, who looks like Colonel Blimp, who is fatter than they want to be?

Such revelation might be accompanied by feelings of self - rejection, discontent, or, even disgust for who we are, to a very deep level. It can feel like we are in an *identity crisis.* So we begin to contemplate change.

This is where people come up with instructions to themselves in their brain. Usually they go something like, `I ought to lose weight', `I wish I was thinner', `I need to tone up', `I really ought to try and be more like a willow and less like a wombat.'

If you've ever done this before, and yet are still reading this book, then you will know that something hasn't worked. To be more precise, *you* haven't worked at what you're doing for exactly the reason that it is far too much like hard work. So your change process hasn't yet fitted with the person that you are and, importantly, the person that you want to be. You haven't been fully motivated, and you haven't been fully congruent with your personal identity.

So this time, how about paying full attention to the question of exactly *why* you want to change your shape or lose weight? Consider, for a moment, what is really important to *you* about being the `right' body shape.

Do you like to think of yourself as healthy or unhealthy, fit or unfit? Or is it for you more about slim or fat, or toned or flabby? Maybe it might be strong or weak, high energy or pooped out.

These are just some ideas. But it's important that you *know* why you want to be healthy, fit, or slim, and what this means to you. In this book, you won't find a chart that tells you a stick insect weight to height ratio. Such charts often seem to suggest that we should be the weight of a stick insect, not helpful. You *will* find lots of encouragement to enjoy the body that you have and work well with it to feel at home with yourself. So you need to decide what is the most important thing to you about becoming the realistic shape and size that you can be!

Because, you know, not everyone is who they seem. Not many people know this, but when those seven dwarves found Snow White out in the forest, she was really upset that her perfect size and looks seemed to be so important for other people, and had caused such jealousy for her step mother. For Snow White, appreciating that her body worked well was all that she wanted. Grumpy, on the other hand, was actually really well worked out but he was grumpy because he could never reach his idea of a perfect shape. Happy was actually a little on the chubby side, but had no physical ailments and just every day appreciated himself for exactly who he was, and was known for his contentment and personality; while Sleepy had no weight issues but did wish now and then that he had more *energy* in his body.

You need to consider who you will *be* when you change your body shape, and how people will describe you - this is Snow White, she's really into long walks in the forest and loves to lift heavy baskets, enjoys the feeling of being strong; this is Happy, he's a very balanced person who is really comfortable with his weight and loves himself; this is Grumpy, he's very fit but never indulges in his favourite food.

So, who do you want to be? What will be your new shape identity?

And when you achieve your changes, when you look in your mirror, and ask yourself `mirror, mirror, on the wall, who is the fairest of them all', what do you really want the answer to be?

❖   `You are, you gorgeous creature, because you look so slim.'

❖   `You are, you lovely person, because your body works and you can tweak it however you want to.'

❖   `You are, you gorgeous creature, because you are relaxed, comfortable, and just as you want to be.'

It's only when you truly know who you want to be, and why, that you can successfully create the right goals in terms of this whole area of weight, shape and size – and you will.

You decide!

Do you want to be the narcissistic person who measures happiness by the size of a thigh but whose frown lines are getting just that little bit deeper with the effort of it all, or do you want to use that mirror as a quick check mechanism, as, deep down, you become comfortable with the marvellous machine that is your body!

There is a nice little saying that we find useful to end this chapter, and it goes like this:

It's not what you think you are – it's what you *think*- you are.

So whatever you do think, make sure that what you're thinking fits with the values that are dear to you, and be the person that you truly want to be.

Doing the following exercises can be extremely useful to engage your brain and body to make desired changes. Grab that pen and paper if it helps!

Name 5 characteristics of yourself that you really like.

1.
2.
3.
4.
5.

Now name 5 that perhaps you like less

1.
2.
3.
4.
5.

Now read each one out loud, while looking into a mirror.

Now tell yourself what is useful or good about all of those characteristics.

Look through this list and decide for yourself what is really the most useful or important scale to rate your body against – what matters most?

❖ Your opinion of yourself, others opinion of you?
❖ Having a body that works well or a body that feels deprived?
❖ Feeling in control, out of control?
❖ Feeling fit, feeling unfit?
❖ Feeling attractive, feeling unattractive?

When you know, write yourself one statement that encapsulates why you want to manage your weight effectively, in terms of who you are.
For example, you might say

I want to be a person who is fit, attractive and energetic,
Confident and not needing other people's approval.

Find the statement that describes the identity that you want to become.

I want to be.............

Now go through your statement of want and take out the extra words, making it shorter. So, in our example, we might take out the verbs and small words, and change it to

Fit, attractive, energetic, confident, person.

The words you come up with are the qualities that you want **to embed in your future identity** as your weight manager.

Now, what words might you use if you were **branding** your new identity, as if in a book title or on an advert?
Our example could become:

Fit, feisty, focused and fabulous!

When you do this for yourself, now you have something easy to remember, something fun that describes who you want to be. Write this down, pin it up even, pop it in your diary. You might even want to add a photo or a `logo' – remember, this is who you are and want to be.

This is what weight management achieves for you ☺

ALADDIN AND HIS MAGIC LAMP

THE ART OF CREATING YOUR GOALS

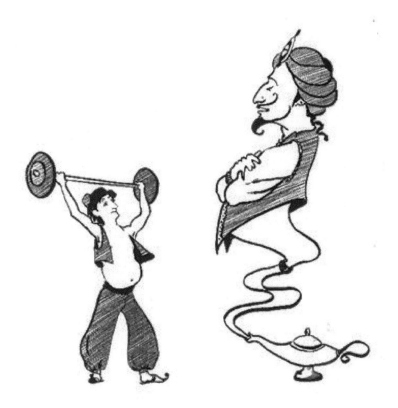

Do any of you remember the story of Aladdin and his magic lamp? Or would any of you like to own a magic lamp? You know the kind that you polish, and when you do, out pops a genie, ready to grant you any wish you want?

Fabulous! Well, imagine that you have such a lamp, and that you could wish for *anything you wanted* to in relation to your size, shape and weight. What would it be?

People often think that they wish to be a certain size, a certain shape, a certain weight. They have a fixed idea born of all sorts of experiences and messages. And now that genie has puffed up into your life and you can have that wish –

Woohoo!

And you can spend a lot of time wishing that things could change – and yet little time considering a really rich picture of what it is that you want them to change *to*.

In this section of the programme, now is the time to get to grips with the answer to a key question. This is the answer which, once you get it absolutely right, will propel you beyond the pivotal point of no return.

It's simple: if you're not happy with your body weight or size, then:

WHAT DO YOU WANT INSTEAD?

Because if you don't yet know the answer, then it's probably not much use thinking what to do next. Should you go to the gym, cut your calories, take up fell walking, do Pilates? If you don't know what you want, then any of these strategies are all a bit of a waste of time.

The first time that the Genie swished magnificently to his full size to grant Aladdin's wishes, he was very excited. A new Master – fabulous. He bowed accordingly.

'*Master, I am the genie of the lamp, and I can grant you three wishes! Anything at all – what will it be?*'

Aladdin grinned, and blinked.

'*Wow, my own genie. To be honest, I'm a bit fed up just now. So, let's see, everyone says I should be a bit thinner, and I wouldn't mind finding myself a nice princess, and maybe, erm, I probably ought to join a gym.*'

Genie looked at him, disappointed. What a ditherer! Here he was, with this fantastic opportunity, and Aladdin just hadn't given his wishes the thought they deserved. He wafted into Aladdin's face.

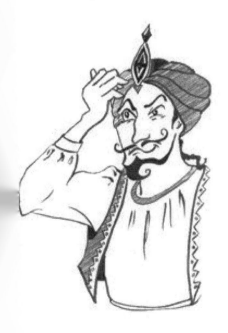

'*Yah boo to you, Sir! Come back when you know what you really wish for!*'

And, with that, he snuck right back into the safety and warmth of the lamp.

Let's put it another way. How many of you have ever had a problem in your life? And when you've had a problem, what's the first thing you do – you ask yourself `what am I going to *do* about it?'

And so you move straight to a solution.

With weight, people do it all the time. Some of *us* have – bet you have too.

`I want to lose a stone/10 kilos. So I'm going on the high protein diet.'

`I want to be slim. So I'm going to fast once a week.'

`I want to be a size 10, or a 36 inch waist. So I've joined a gym.'

Okay, a reasonable start – you have a rough idea of where you want to get to, and some ideas of how. However, this is not enough. These answers, if you are not careful - and we might suggest that it is useful to be extremely full of care toward yourself - are just statements of intent, often subconsciously littered with `should', `ought', `have to', `need to.'

Sometimes, we even have an unhelpful statement hidden in our brain, such as `but I know I'll find it hard', `but I can't seem to', `but I'll never do it while Fred will only eat chips and mush.' These hidden thoughts might leap out to justify our behaviour if we don't quite achieve what we want.

And then we find we really *haven't* used the power of the Genie; instead we've got sidetracked by the cry of `New Lamps for Old', but haven't really thought in depth as to what that new lamp needs to be like, in order to get us the wishes that we really want to fulfill.

In Mirror, Mirror we explore some of the perceptions, thoughts and feelings you might have about who you are, and who you really want to be. So now, let's put some flesh (well toned, of course!) on the bones of this idea – let's get specific about what you want instead. This is not only about how you want to *look* when you are the `perfect' shape, but how you want to *feel,* what you want to be *telling* yourself instead of what you're telling yourself now, and what all of these things together will really achieve for you.

It's easy to begin to get a sense of `what do you want instead?' Let's just sit and ponder, for a moment, what might happen when you've rubbed your beautiful personal magic lamp. Instead of any old Genie springing out to help you, imagine that, to your surprise and pleasure, a genie in your own image pops out – a full size image of a future you, the size and shape that you want to be. Standing there, picture perfect. Take a good look at yourself. Notice how you look, what colours you are wearing, the expression on your face. When you've had a really good peruse all around, take a mental step inside that image. Notice what posture you are taking,: notice your breathing.; notice how you feel, when you become the person that you wish to be. Imagine that `you' in social situations, private situations, work situations, moving along your chosen roads feeling really good about the body you have, however it may be.

Good, isn't it?

And when you imagine that you are the weight, shape and size you want to be, the future you, ask yourself,

What does that achieve for me?

Often, we find that shape change achieves more confidence, more relaxation, a degree of comfort. You are all different, so really think about what these changes will give you more of, and what they will release you from.

So. Back to now. As you contemplate your change, and just before you make plans, a few more things to consider. You may wonder how you will feel in the future if you do not change your shape and size, get rid of your dissatisfaction, manage to wear different clothes, or have the energy that you want. What is that like?

In other words, what happens if you don't make the changes?

Because people often say, don't they, I can't seem to lose weight, I can't resist temptation —and that's right, you can always *not* do things if you choose.

Or you can choose that you can.

And it's important to recognize that in order to achieve more of something, you may need to let some things go. Walking might replace a habitual TV. programme. Meals out may be less appealing. Change brings consequences, so it's good to know what they will be.

So consider what it is that you want from *your* personal Genie, and what that will achieve for you. And when you know this *ultimate* wish, you need to remember it in some way, write it down somewhere, embed it in your head, or put a post it on your computer, on your fridge – whatever it is for you. You can go through this process again in the Application section at the end of this chapter if you would like to.

When you know clearly what it is you want, it helps to make your goal, compelling. You need to be clear that your **want** is exactly that, not an *ought*, a *should*, or a *might*, - far too wishy washy!

Let's recap. Now you know what you want instead of what you have now. You know what this achieves for you, and you know what you will be seeing, hearing and feeling when you get there. You know what might be the consequences of making such change, and of making no change.

Now in order to nail this on, there are some principles that we know about goals which will increase your chance of reaching and sustaining them. They need to be **specific** – do you want to make small changes, big changes or medium sized changes - you need to know. And **how will you know when you've got there?** Remember what you will be feeling, seeing, thinking, hearing and saying. How will you

measure success: are you going to use a tape measure, a weighing scale, an item of clothing, or something different as your barometer.

Is your goal **appropriate**? If you are dissatisfied with your shape, losing one cm from your left thigh is unlikely to give you the achievement you want! Size matters! Equally, your goal needs to be within your control and within your resources. It is not likely that at the age of 60 your ideal or achievable body shape and weight will be the same as it was at 20. And the genetic aspects of your shape (pear, apple, banana – banana??!!) will rarely be fully changeable, unless you choose surgery as one of your strategies.

And you need a time frame – if you tell me that you will lose 2 stones by next Thursday, or you tell me that you want to lose weight, but without an end in mind – then your goal will not be compelling. By when will you have the changes that you want?

Finally, and crucially, your goal needs to be **compelling**. **Does it excite you?** You need to be talking about what you *will* be doing, what you *are* doing, not what you're *trying* to be doing. In fact ban the word `trying' from your vocabulary! Remember, weight management is something that you **want** and **can do**.

By now, you are learning how to stack up your compelling goal – and now your personal genie might be taking some notice. Just as Aladdin did when

Aladdin had put in the work on his goals and rubbed the magic lamp once more. Out swished the Genie, bowing once again.

'Master, what a pleasure to see you. How can I help?'

Aladdin grinned sheepishly.

'Hello, Genie, excellent to see you. I am going to lose 7 kilos over a three month period, because then I will be more confident. This will be fab, because then I will enjoy being able to wear my favourite clothes, and I will feel really good with myself while I get to know that gorgeous Princess. Feeling confident will help me down the bazaar, as well, and I've got a great vision of how I will look, know how my posture will be, and how great I feel. I just can't wait!'

Genie beamed from ear to ear, pulled excitedly at the ends of his moustache, clapped his hands.

'Wow, you are one clear and

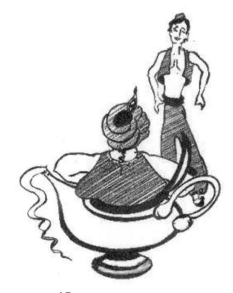

motivated lamp owner – the best I've ever had! I'm really excited to give you that support, and will be here beside you to illuminate the way – and then when you've got that far, you'll *still* have two wishes left! Doesn't leave much for me to do – hope I don't get fat and lazy sitting in that lamp!'

When you **identify what you want** instead of what you have now, **imagine fully** what that **outcome** will achieve for you, *and* rehearse how **great** that will be, you will experience an exciting shift. You will quickly learn to enjoy each step of achieving your goals, rather than `working' towards enjoyment at the end. You might surprise yourself by discovering that it is really satisfying to eat only what you want to in the quantities that you choose, and to relish moving your body in whichever way you want. You can also have the pleasure of identifying and reaching significant milestones to celebrate and enhance you motivation.

By making these good decisions about what you *want*, you are preparing to succeed. This means that you will easily generate precise and effective action plans.

And that's another story!

SUGGESTED EXERCISES

Notice how you are phrasing what you want before you begin to take action. Try the following statements out loud, while watching yourself in a mirror, and notice which feels, looks and sounds most compelling.

- ❖ I *ought* to lose weight
- ❖ I *need* to lose weight
- ❖ I *intend* to lose weight
- ❖ I'm *trying* to lose weight
- ❖ I *want* to lose weight
- ❖ I **will** lose weight

Maybe weight is not your thing, maybe it's shape, inches, fitness, maybe it's maintaining your status quo - replace the instruction and follow the same exercise.

When you identify your compelling statement, write it down.

I will………..

Then repeat it out loud, *I will…*

Next, take yourself through the following questions in relation to your weight management. Give yourself time to write down your answers and consider as many of the questions as you find helpful..

What, **specifically,** in terms of your weight management, do you want instead of what you have now?

- ❖ What will this **achieve** for you?
- ❖ How will you know when you have made the changes you want?
- ❖ How will other people know?
- ❖ When you succeed, what will be happening that isn't happening now?
- ❖ What will not be happening?
- ❖ In what ways will you be feeling different?
- ❖ In what ways might you be behaving differently?
- ❖ How could your changes affect your work /your home life/your leisure time?
- ❖ What will you be thinking that you're not thinking now?
- ❖ What will you have stopped thinking?
- ❖ What would an average day/week/month look like?
- ❖ What might you have to give up?
- ❖ What might it cost those near to you?
- ❖ How will it benefit you?
- ❖ Those near to you?
- ❖ If you do nothing, what will it cost you?
- ❖ Those near to you?
- ❖ How would `no change' benefit you?
- ❖ With all of this knowledge in mind, by when do you want to have achieved your weight management goal?

CINDERELLA

DISCOVERING STRENGTHS AND RESOURCES

I *shall* go to the ball! How often have we heard or made that declaration of triumph in our lives? Good old Cinders – she's the real rags to riches story, the girl who got exactly what she wanted against all the odds.

How capable are *we* of achieving what we really want and how do we do that? What qualities and resources are available to us that we can harness and use to our greatest advantage?

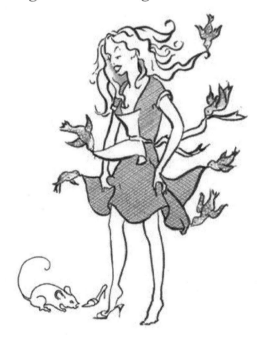

Consider how resourceful Cinderella was in her bid to get to the ball *despite* the stepmother from hell and the ugly sisters. Not to mention having no suitable

49

dress to wear, masses of housework to complete and all the rest (I'm sure you remember the story.) Pretty resourceful, we would say!

We, like Cinderella, have all experienced times in our lives when we are pushed and catapulted into action and miraculously, from nowhere it seems, we find incredible inner strengths and resources that drive us forward.

Sound familiar? We imagine so!

How fantastic would it be to be able to access these resources whenever we want to, enabling us to use them in a proactive, knowing way rather than reactively and blindly?

We all have incredible strengths and resources available to us: it's just that we don't always use them to the greatest potential. The trick is *getting to know them well* so that we are able to use them with intention that serves our ends.

Let's consider Cinderella's example. She clearly gained a good sense and knowledge of *her* resources, strengths and skills, with excellent results – not only did she fit beautifully into the glass slipper when it mattered most, she also caught Prince Charming from under the noses of her wicked siblings ☺.

It may be helpful to think about some of the capabilities that she drew on. The first thing that comes to mind is the team she had behind her success – external resources. Before meeting the Fairy Godmother, Cinderella was very much in the pre-contemplation stage of change, accepting her lot, as the underdog at the beck and call of her hideous sisters and step mother; she never considered that it could be any different. Then along came that Fairy Godmother with her magic, and she orchestrated the whole show. Cinderella moved swiftly through to action planning changes once she believed that she had the support to do it.

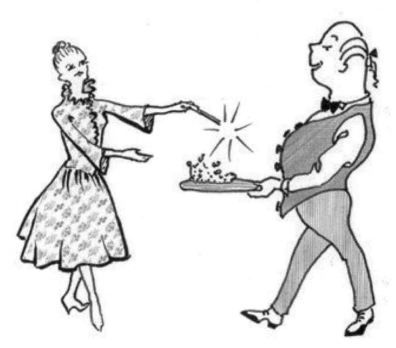

Buttons, faithful and loyal, was busy in the background supporting the show, yet Cinders did not always realize that. And let's not forget the seamstress birds that made that exquisite dress - *and* the mice that pulled the coach that took her to the Ball and got everything into action. The greatest gift that Cinders gained from the team was the belief that it was *possible* to do and be something different!

What do you imagine that *your* capabilities might be?

Take a moment to think about who is around in your life that may be an active supporter on your quest to reach and maintain the weight and shape that you want to be. It may be a close friend or family member; it may be a colleague or a professional. Or is there someone you see as a role model, someone you admire for what they have achieved- what could you learn or take from them? Are there any available groups that you think may be of benefit to you, for example a slimming group, exercise group of some kind, or social group? Think widely here and access what works for you.

Cinders also used her internal resources. No-one could deny her determination and will; she completed all the household tasks that had been deliberately set to interfere with any chance of her attending the Ball. Not to mention her bold behaviour when trying on the glass slipper in front of her unknowing, bewildered and furious family.

What of your determination and will? When have you been able to use these before? Consider how you might engage with these inner qualities so that you are able to use them wisely and achieve what you desire.

We all truly admired Cinders' assertive self. There she was, faced with such bullies, yet in her own way (accessing her internal strength) she stood up to them to meet her needs and desires. Might there be times that you will need to draw on some of your own assertiveness to enable you to tackle those people who may attempt to hijack your success? You recognise the ones, 'oh go on, a couple of biscuits won't hurt,' or 'forget the gym today; let's just go for a coffee instead!' It can be very helpful for you to rehearse in advance how you will choose to respond to these situations.

What about all the knowledge and skills that you have to draw on, and what additional knowledge might you need?

Let's face it; we all know the basics of weight loss or gain. It's a simple principle. If what we take in (our eating and drinking) exceeds what we use in energy, we gain weight! If what we take in is less than the amount of energy we use, then we lose weight. With this premise in mind, if we're not the weight we want to be, we just need to shift the balance.

Simple! Well, yes. However, do you need to learn more *detail* around this to help you on your way? Is your understanding about different food and drink types *enough*, knowing what to avoid or limit for example? Different people have different knowledge bases. Where might you access additional knowledge if you choose?

How did Cinders find her way to the Ball?

Another way of shifting the balance is to use exercise -burning off some of the energy taken in, which also has the benefit of strengthening our hearts. We know that although we never saw Cinderella in the gym, she was incredibly active with all the household tasks, unlike her lazy and overweight sisters.

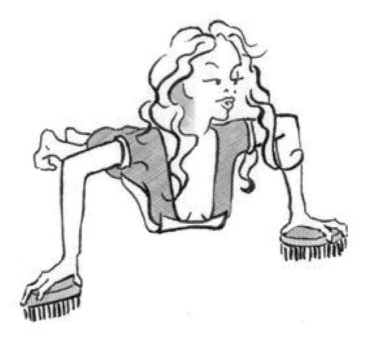

What activity might you choose that will help here? What might you enjoy and easily fit into your life? Do you need any additional knowledge and expertise regarding exercise, about how much to do to make the appropriate difference? Who might be able to help with that, and are you able to access and accept such help? After all, accessing and accepting help worked for Cinderella. Without it, she wouldn't have made the Ball or got to marry the Prince, so worth remembering!

There are many external resources out there, and no doubt you can push yourself to think widely about the whole range available to you.

As well as knowing what resources might aid you, it is also necessary to be aware of what is *not* so helpful, and to identify things that can get in the way. Some of these might be beliefs and behaviours, which we explore elsewhere, and some may be triggers in our environment - `see Haagen-Dazs, must scoff', that sort of thing. Why is it helpful to know what might be unhelpful – simple, because to be forewarned is to be forearmed.

The idea is that if you know about potential obstacles you can prepare and ward them off (as Cinderella did with the ugly sisters), using the capabilities you have available to you. So what else would you like to have or need? Think resourcefully here! If you know you're going to that Haagen-Dazs zone, plan now for whether or not you'll indulge. If you decide to, then work out what other food you might leave out that day, or what additional activity you do – use your inner capability to plan. Or if you choose to say no to that particular temptation, use your internal resources of self discipline and assertiveness. The capabilities are all there – bring them to mind, identify them, rehearse the life you will have if you use them to the full.

Perhaps you know other people as well as Cinders who have been successful, what can you identify in them which may be helpful to add to your collection? Take a good look around you.

Spending time thinking about the strengths and resources you currently access frequently, and those you want to access, *before* embarking on your weight loss journey, will ensure you are well prepared and armed with the necessary tools to support you. Pre planning before action is essential, because remember that it's only worth doing what works!

Brilliant, isn't it – you can become your very own Fairy Godmother, releasing the magic which is always within yourself to remember how very many resources you already have, what a vast amount of knowledge to call on, which, once accessed will get you wherever you want to go.

SUGGESTED EXERCISES

Grab paper and pen and find a comfortable, quiet spot.

Think back to that time when you have changed something in your life, ideally around weight loss if you have tried this before.

How did you do it?

What internal resources and strengths do you have which helped you on your way? These may be your knowledge or qualities for example. We are hoping for a long list here!

When you feel you have logged them all, ask yourself to add just 2 more. Think about what someone close to you would say your strengths were. Are they right?

Add them to the list!

Now we want you to think of external resources. What do you have available to you? Think widely here, as once identified these are going to aid your success on this particular journey. You might find the following prompts useful.

- ❖ People?
- ❖ Places?
- ❖ IT resources –groups, programmes, information?
- ❖ Slimming Clubs?
- ❖ Television?
- ❖ Distraction – Reading, Walking, Talking, Meditation, Relaxation (list is endless here)?
- ❖ Books (This book for example – hmm, maybe that ought to be top of the list?)
- ❖ Magazines?

Beware of those negative 'resources' – saboteurs!

Identify those resources that are NOT so trustworthy, like, in Cinders' case, the ugly sisters! Some **people** will want you, even encourage you, to fall off the wagon… 'Oh don't worry, why bother you look fine anyway!'

Sometimes it's your **own thoughts** that can damage your resources - e.g. 'I'm not sure I can do this!' (You know, those annoying self-doubts which it would appear Cinderella didn't have).

Or maybe a **behaviour** that you have … 'whenever I have any alcohol I have to have........'

Finally, it may be that there are things that you don't yet have that are important for your success. You may be capable of running but you don't own any decent trainers yet.

Whatever it is, identify the saboteurs now and counter them with resources and capabilities.

THE HARE AND THE TORTOISE

CHOOSING BELIEFS FOR A CHANGE

*The Hare and the Tortoise i*s one of Aesop's famous fables. It tells the tale of what happens when the boastful Hare and determined Tortoise enter a race together. Hare believes that he will win easily, so stops for a snooze on the way, while Tortoise believes that slow and steady wins the day, and proceeds

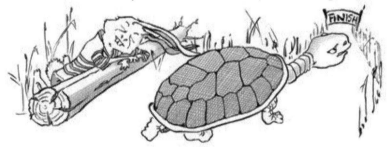

to overtake the sleeping Hare and win the race. It would be easy to think that it is about the notion that slow achievement is more effective than the quick fix. We agree with the wisdom of that notion, *and* we add a slightly different tack.

We believe that what we believe about ourselves, others, and the world in general, has a most powerful effect on everyday life. Our beliefs influence everything.

So using beliefs to our advantage in everything we do can make us masters of our own destiny. Because although we believe that life is not a rehearsal, we also know that life *is* a rehearsal – we rehearse in our heads all the time. So let's rehearse using the beliefs that serve us well.

It's a strange thing, a belief. Some of us have beliefs that have been instilled in us since our childhood. Some of them are cultural and may stay with us forever. Some others can be easily changed or modified to suit our ever changing life, lifestyle, and the world around us.

Aesop's Tortoise, of course, knew all this very well indeed. Whereas Hare had not a clue. Until after the race had been run, and he and Tortoise were lying on the grass together recovering from the effort it all.

`Tortoise', said Hare, a little perplexed. `How did you do that?'

Tortoise extended his neck – slowly. Chewed lazily on a blade of grass.

`Well, very easily, actually, Hare. My mother, bless her shell, taught me to believe that determination is deeply rewarding, and that beating others isn't as important as doing your best. And I believe that, always do your best. I don't know whether you'd agree, Hare, but I also believe that you can do most things that you really want to. And if you want real long lasting change, then slow and steady is more effective than exhausting spurts.'

Hare was mystified.

`But even so, I'm so fast when I want to be. So what did I do wrong?'

Tortoise blinked hard.

`Well, I think you looked at the wrong things. You chose a disabling belief, that fast is best. You have a wonderful skill of being able to run and to use the energy of your body. Now if you focus on *that*, believing that it's great to enjoy your body for your own sake, taking pleasure in the feeling of your body moving, you would do well. Instead of that, you were focused on the race, believed you were better than me, and so you became complacent.'

Hare's ears twitched at that. He knew the Tortoise to be right, but was none too pleased with himself.

`But I suppose that I'm worried about changing my approach in case I lose all the fun of my personality.'

Tortoise blinked.

`Then you must change your belief, Hare, and realize that all it takes to get to where you want to is to change your beliefs – and then you can change some of your habits without really changing your personality at all.'

Hare nodded, accepting the wisdom of Tortoise's words.

`I believe this to be true. But how do I change my beliefs, Tortoise?'

Tortoise nodded, a half smile playing on his lips.

`Far be it from me to suggest that it can be easy, Hare, but try this to begin with. Think about what's important to you – your values. Like `it's good to value your body', for example. Then picture your body doing the things you want it to – because you know, Hare, mind and body are the same system. Imagine you are capable of anything, and notice what you would be doing if that were true. Know that you are capable of finishing, and make your body and mind work the best you can for you – not for anyone else, just for you. Make yourself in your mind's eye as fit and as successful as you want to be.'

Hare was beginning to get it, nodding away. `And then you can do it', he said, almost to himself.

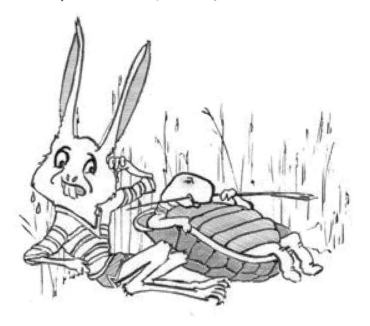

So, we believe that not all beliefs have to be true. We also believe that some untrue beliefs can be helpful. Our advice is therefore to **choose the beliefs that serve you best!**

When you apply this principle to weight management, you will need to hold certain beliefs that will sustain you in that pursuit. You may also need to lose some disabling beliefs. In our experience, those of you who choose to believe that you can shape your own destiny tend to succeed in … shaping your own destiny☺. Those of you who believe that you are strong will behave as if you are strong. You get the idea - you can choose to believe *whatever helps you most* to embed in your brain and heart that you really can achieve the weight and size that you want.

So, you may be wondering how you can train yourself to embed some of those powerful beliefs which you know to be helpful.

Well let's stop and ponder. Firstly, you know that by buying this book you have already started the change process. This is great. At the beginning of his particular journey, poor old Hare doesn't even *know* he needs to change, and Tortoise – well, he's just a Tortoise.

To progress beyond this first step, imagine what life could be like if you were able to identify some of the current beliefs that you hold which are disabling, for example, `I get so hungry', `losing weight is horrible because you have to be hungry', `I'm helpless', `it's in my genes' (or, in the case of the chubbier thighed, it's in my jeans☺)

These beliefs might have been helpful in the past, as you might have had good reason for not yet letting them go. If you are now ready to take full charge of your weight management, you do need now to acknowledge their contribution to making you the person that you are, and mentally bin them.

Next, consider how it might be if you admit that you *can* change; admit you *could* have better beliefs in your head. Then you can identify which beliefs would be more helpful. For example, you might choose to believe that you really *can* take charge of your eating and energy levels while feeling good. Wow! Then you could commit to changing the thoughts in your head, and believing that this is a really powerful and helpful way to go. It is liberating to put ideas and beliefs into your head which will enable you to think more positively, and to believe that you can most definitely get to your own finishing post.

So, choose your beliefs wisely, and begin to imagine how it might be if you adopt them daily. Some people like to record their more helpful beliefs in some way – writing them down, putting them on their i-Pods and Pads, making a dream board, make up a mantra – whatever works for you. The more you remember the powerful useful beliefs, then the easier it is to reassure yourself and encourage yourself if that old Tortoise seems a bit too slow, or retreats into his shell now and then.

Simple, isn't it, how the possibilities become almost endless when you believe that you can change what's in your mind. And when a voice in your mind is telling you things you *don't* want to hear, d'you know what – you can always answer back, and tell the whiney voice of gloom to zip it! Because if you keep on telling yourself the right things, you can keep on doing the things that are right for you.

In the case of the Hare and the Tortoise, the Tortoise achieved his goal, whereas silly old Hare really messed up. He was so complacent, so competitive with others instead of paying attention to his inner and outer self, that he fell asleep.

The great thing was that, as we have revealed here, he then was prepared, just like you, to learn from past mistakes. And, with Tortoise's help, he learned that, as ever, it's not what you think you are – it's what you *think*, you are.

When you admit that you *can* change, you can commit to changing the thoughts in your head. Have a think about some of the following and see if you could lose some beliefs and gain some others! Feel free to add in others on either list.

Lose the unhelpful, such as

❖ I get so hungry I can't bear it
❖ I have a low metabolic rate
❖ It's genetic
❖ I can't leave food on a plate while people starve

Acquire the helpful, such as

❖ I can do anything I want, I can achieve almost anything, and all I need is time and commitment, which I have
❖ I can learn from past attempts and am now wiser about how to get what I want
❖ I am strong
❖ I believe in what I set out to do
❖ I believe in the future, and I enjoy the present
❖ My life and health are important to me
❖ I can be realistic and optimistic
❖ When I think positively about the best outcome I am likely to succeed
❖ I am a person who will get where I want to be

- ❖ I deserve all that I work toward
- ❖ Changing shape form or weight is possible for me
- ❖ I am going to succeed now
- ❖ I am someone who sticks to the programme
- ❖ I am as able as anyone else
- ❖ I choose my own destiny

Write down for yourself the three most powerful beliefs that you could possibly have to support you in managing your weight.

1.
2.
3.

You might want to record them somehow – you choose which way is right for you.....

- ❖ write them down

- ❖ say them to yourself

- ❖ put them to music

- ❖ have them on your iPod, computer screensaver, fridge door, car windscreen, TV screen and so on

Live everyday as if these beliefs are true; revisit them every time you feel the need for reassurance and encouragement.

We know from time to time you might let a less than optimistic thought escape through your lips or inside your head....get back on track with a few **antidotes**. For example notice the beginning of the sentence below, and notice how the added words after the dots neutralise the damage of the first part:

❖ It's not happening…**yet.**
❖ Oh dear, it's a nightmare, a disaster, awful …**and tomorrow is a new day for a new start**.
❖ I knew I couldn't…**and yet I know I can and will persist.**
❖ It's so hard… **and those hard things get easier and easier with each successful step.**
❖ I'm so hungry….**at the moment, and I can cope with that, perhaps I need to plan better.**
❖ I deserve a treat…**yes I do and I'll have a good one …when *I* say so, not when hat silly whiney voice in my head tells me to!**

BEAUTY AND THE BEAST

FINDING BEHAVIOURS THAT WORK

In the story of Beauty and The Beast, Beast was

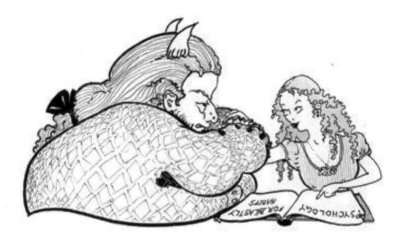

desperate for Beauty, and believed that he could never have her. If only the Beast had beauty, then Beauty could be had. Beauty on the other hand was much more impressed by the behaviour of the beast than his looks.

It is little known, but Beauty was a trained psychologist and an expert in behaviour change. Isn't that amazing? Even less well known is that she helped the beast change by using a few bits of inside knowledge, and a purely psychological approach. Despite his awful shape and general ugliness, Beauty became very fond of the beast, suspecting that his appearance was not all his fault, nor his whole identity. She had also noticed that despite keeping her captive, he treated her very well. Beauty wanted to be free, and yet she could not leave the beast in such a state.

Well, that's not so surprising is it: after all she was a generous and helpful person, and that was part of her beauty.

Just like you perhaps?

One of the things that Beauty was heard to say to Beast was:

`If you keep on doing what you've always done you will keep on getting what you've always got.'

At first, Beast didn't understand this, but sometimes, as you know, you have to repeat things to understand them, and so he did. Then he eventually got the message. *And* even added on the next bit for himself – `so to *get* something different, I need to *do* something different.'

Beauty was really smart. She knew that the beast was very strong, and that to tame him she had to use all her powers and influence. She knew that on first acquaintance Beast was somewhat unpleasant to look at: part of that was that he was so fat she could barely see his features and expression, and part was that he was so full of grease that he had unpleasant spots and blackheads. So she began to wonder how to enable change.

She noticed that Beast had adopted a few nasty habits. For example, he often ate late at night. Sometimes when he ate she wondered whether in fact he really just needed a cuddle. She also noticed that sometimes he was nearly trembling when he ate and then went for sugary buns, causing her to wonder if he had gone too long between meals, lowering his blood sugar levels. Sometimes he seemed to eat out of habit, say when it was 4 o'clock – time for tea! Or because he was watching a certain TV programme. And often he would eat to give himself a treat, which was fine, but he did have an awful *lot* of treats, and on occasion Beauty had heard Beast saying that eating chocolate in the car didn't count because food has no calories

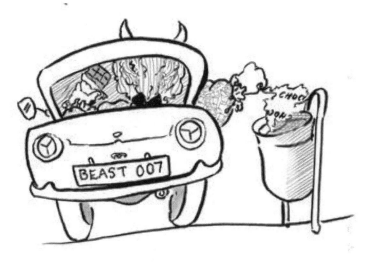

inside a moving vehicle! Beauty also noticed that Beast did not drink water regularly, and wondered if on occasion he ate when really he needed hydration – perhaps confusing thirst with hunger.

Despite being such a well trained analyst, it was not at first apparent to Beauty that the beast was completely besotted with her. Actually, he was putty in her hands, so once she'd made a mental record of how he was doing what he did, and once she realised how motivated to change he was, she was able to give him some tips.

71

'Beast', she would say, 'I know you think that if you swallow food quickly it doesn't count, and that starving yourself will help you lose weight, but you are wrong.'

This really got his attention.

'It's much more important that you begin to understand your own behaviour.'

'Really?' Beast blinked hard at Beauty. 'I'll get prepared to listen, then.'

'Well', said Beauty, 'to be beautiful, inside and out, it is important to behave beautifully. You need to identify what sorts of behaviours are keeping you from achieving your goals. Begin to notice carefully what you eat and when, when you eat things you don't really enjoy. Notice what kind of foods you eat, and how well planned your meals are. Notice whether or not you exercise. More than anything, notice if what goes in to your body is more or less than the energy you use. And check your grease consumption – you'll never lose your spots if you live on tubs of lard. Look closely at your own behaviour and sometimes let others give you some feedback.'

Beast blinked gratefully.

'Until you arrived, I realise I had been hiding away, and no one had ever been kind or honest enough to give me that helpful feedback.'

Beauty told Beast that there are no ways of **not** behaving. When you stop doing something, you don't leave a vacuum, you have to put something in its place. This is perhaps why when you give something up, you replace it with something else.

The trick is to begin to realise that you are *never* giving up something good – this implies a deprivation. The only thing that you are giving up is feeling dissatisfied or trapped. It is more useful to consider yourself as replacing an undesirable behaviour with something that is desirable – something you *want to keep*, not something that will take some more will power to get rid of in the future.

You may be thinking that some of this is obvious, and it is; yet sometimes we are in such a rush to change things that we don't remember to give the process of change enough thought or preparation.

So, Beauty believed that Beast needed to be more observant about how his behaviour impacted on his goal, as do you. He needed to be more *accurate* in how he measured his habitual behaviour.

'Oh Beast,' said Beauty, 'you *must* take more control over what you put in your mouth, and lots of your eating habits.'

The beast decided to change many of his habits to healthier ones such as only eating when he was hungry, thinking carefully about what he ate, making sure that he enjoyed his food, and stopping when he was full. He also learned to consider how food might feel inside him half an hour after he'd eaten it - could he choose foods that *give* energy over foods that take energy to digest?

Once he started to make these changes, he nudged closer to beauty day by day.

You can see that these behaviours are really easy to change once we acknowledge them, and that you really can follow Beast's example. We don't know which of the behaviour changes you want to begin with, or which is the easiest and quickest one to change first, but we know that you do!

Once begun, you'll notice other aspects and habits which might have an impact on your behaviours, and which might impact on your ability to achieve your goal.

Personally, one of us hates the thought of exercise simply for the sake of exercise. Not everyone shares that perception, and it is evidenced that if you want to make changes that are permanent, you may need to increase your activity levels. One of our number loves exercise precisely for the sake of exercise, and the achievement and self esteem that

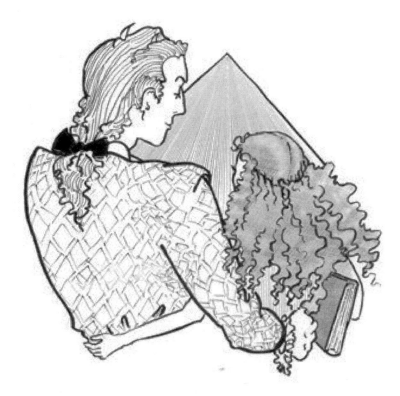

comes with fitness. Another of us likes a mix, some 'for its own sakes', some which combines responsibilities such as dog walking. And the one of our number who dislikes the thought of exercise for exercise's sake, really enjoys activities such as chasing a golf ball about, making love, making something for the shed, going to dancing lessons, digging the garden. Remember Cinders? Never made it to the gym, yet always busy. There's more than one way to get active.

For us, and we suspect you too, the trick is to find activity that you enjoy. Enjoyment motivates you to get out of the armchair and boost that metabolic rate a tad. Exercise must be rewarding, as Beauty made clear to Beast. She explained to him that punishing yourself does *not* help you become more motivated, so make sure that any exercise you choose is interesting, and rewarding. Then you will go back and do it again.

Beauty also encouraged Beast to remember to build in treats along the way - 'If you want that bar of chocolate, Beast my friend, then have it ...but maybe only after you have done something physically engaging; or maybe take two squares a day instead of two blocks.'

She was right, wasn't she, because we all know, that changing behaviours grudgingly and without reward won't work. More useful to choose a pattern that will.

We come back to the fact that once you know how, changing your behaviour is one of the most important and easiest things to do. So how do you start, and how do you maintain the change?

Well, Beauty very cleverly reminded Beast to remember the change cycle. And it goes like this:

❖   Notice that you want something different about your shape or weight
❖   Discover what you want to be different and what this will achieve
❖   Begin to chart or note your eating and activity behaviours
❖   Get a clear idea about what behaviours you want to change
❖   Find suitable ways, means, ideas, strategies
❖   Let success build on success, and reward here and there
❖   If you lapse, get back on track as soon as possible. Have a think about what behaviours need tweaking or reinforcing, and re-instate the new behaviours. It's unlikely that you will need to go right back to the beginning, as you have already had success.
❖   And if you do – then just tell yourself okay, that was fun, and store your learnings inside for next time.

We might remind you that the tale of Beauty and the Beast concludes when her tears of love for him flowed onto his face as he prostrated himself before her. And then he turned into the Prince of his dreams. The power of love.

So remember, as we've said before, **be kind to yourself, for where-ever you go, there you'll be**.

SUGGESTED EXERCISES

Changing your behaviour will be important, because if you keep on doing what you've always done ...you will have no change at all. So do something different!

Remember some hints and ideas to help you change your weight shape or form:

- Eating late at night increases your likelihood to weight gain.
- Notice when you eat for other reasons than hunger
  o just needed a cuddle or reassurance
  o needed an energy boost or craved sugar (he didn't plan meals well)
  o bored
  o thirsty not hungry
  o just out of habit...it's 6 O'clock – time for tea!
  o You deserve a treat (illicit treats can become too much
- Eat only delicious things
- Notice how hungry you are before eating
- Drink when thirsty instead of eating
- Eat only when you really want to
- Eat foods that sustain you, instead of quick fixes
- Do something exciting, interesting, and useful instead of eating
- Become aware of **when** you are eating and what **rituals** you have developed

Exercise using strategies that INTEREST you like:

- ❖ Making love
- ❖ Chasing a golf ball about
- ❖ Household activity such as painting the kitchen, sanding a work surface, laying some tiles, cleaning , gardening, walking to the shops, playing games, using the gym, dancing, swimming – you choose

- ❖ Keep an eye on the calorie in/calorie out equation. We don't advocate obsessive calorie counting, yet it is necessary to know the calories in/calories out equation which underlies weight management

- ❖ Question yourself when you notice there is something in your mouth!
  Did I put it there?
    - ➤ Purposefully?
    - ➤ Deliberately?
    - ➤ Because I am really hungry?
    - ➤ Because I am bored?
    - ➤ Or because it's really delicious and I consciously, and deliberately and carefully decided to eat it!

- ❖ Shop after you have eaten
- ❖ Spend time with people who are supportive to your objectives, not with saboteurs
- ❖ Say what you really mean, and be mean to people who are being beastly to you.

❖ Control some of those beastly thoughts (see The Hare and the Tortoise), to influence your behaviours.
❖ Know your hunger scale, how hungry are you on a scale of 0-10? Only eat at 7 or more, say.
❖ Only have pudding if you fancy it and sometimes have it instead of the main course.

These are all ideas. Having considered them, write down 3 behavioural changes that you can make from now on which will make a significant difference.

1
.
2.

3.

Keep these, alongside your goals, your beliefs and your capabilities, and stack them up to make those moves towards full weight management.

Mary, Mary, quite contrary

CREATING THE RIGHT ENVIRONMENTS

Mary, Mary, quite contrary - how *did* her garden grow?

You know, we are all influenced by our surroundings. In weight management, it becomes crucial to prepare your personal environment to suit your personal needs.

Just as Mary did. She created a lovely little garden, thank you very much, with just whatever she wanted in it to please her, even if it had things in it – silver bells and cockle shells – that might not have been to everybody's taste.

Now then, what a lot of people don't realise, is that Mary didn't create that garden without any support. No indeed, she had a *gardener*. Someone to give her lots of hints and tips.

`Mary,' he said, `the first thing you need to do in your garden is have a good look around and see what needs throwing out. You'll need to dig some stuff up, and take it to the compost. You'll have to cut some stuff back and prune it right down, so that you can grow fresh branches and flowers.'

We move in lots of environments, don't we, which we might need to plan differently or respond to carefully, when making changes for weight management. There's home, work, public, media, natural, events, travel, holiday. All of these places are full of traps, receptacles of bad or unhelpful habits (sneaking into the kitchen to steal that last roast potato from the side, rather than putting it in the bin!); *and* all have the potential to be our allies.

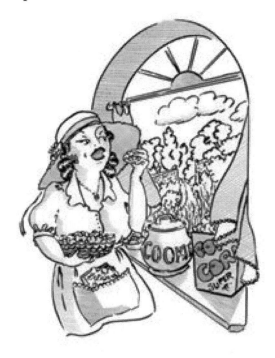

In terms of clearing and pruning, one of the most powerful places to begin is at home. Specifically, cupboards, large and small, built in or free standing, electrical or not. Wardrobes, food cupboards, fridges – even bedside tables!

Before going any further, right now, have a look inside your wardrobe, at least mentally, if not physically. What's in it? - any clothes that you don't wear any more, any that don't fit, any that you really don't feel comfortable in, any that make you look more frightening than fabulous? There is a rule of thumb here – if in doubt throw it out! Your wardrobe needs pruning, because, as any gardener will tell you, cutting back will generate a more healthy growth.

However, it may be that you decide to keep some of the clothes that currently don't fit as motivation to achieving your goal of getting into them once again, that favourite dress or pair of trousers, for example.   If that's so, and if your commitment to change is compelling, then keep it.   However, give yourself a numbers limit on how many items you keep, with only one visible on a daily basis as a measurement bar. Crucially, give yourself a time frame by which you'll fit them, and make it realistic. By all means use clothes this way, as a measurement of success – but beware hanging on to reminders of a past rather than looking to a future. Meanwhile, a key aid to losing weight is to wear only clothes in which you feel the very best that you can feel. There's enough inner turmoil going on without undermining your self confidence even further. Feel good to feel motivated – it really helps.

What about your food cupboards and your fridge –more cream than bream? The fridge of the wibbly wombat, or the fridge of the self determined self-caring person? Enough to feed an army or enough to feed a family and a guest? Food that reflects enjoyment or food that reflects compulsion – go on, dive in, have a look, and be honest. If there are weeds in there, as Mary's gardener would be the first to say, they will keep on rooting down and out so that no new growth can come, and the new you cannot flower – so throw them out!

And the food cupboard.   Tins, packets, whatever it is, if it's wrong for your change, or there's too much of it, clear it out. Create the space to forge your new path.

`So what when I've cleared the space, then,' Mary asked her gardener friend, before beginning the next phase.

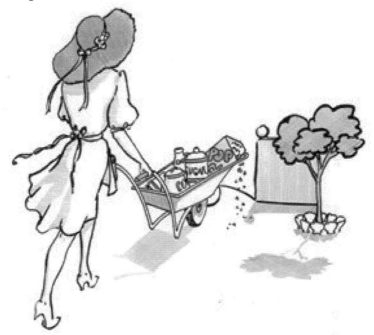

`Well, Mary, you're going to have to just revisit what you want to be doing, and then make sure that you've got the right tools and resources. You'll need ways to plant what you want, and you'll need the right nourishment to make your seeds grow.'

Aha. Tools and resources. Well, in food terms, that can become fairly simple. Foods that give you energy, rather than foods that make you want to fall asleep. Foods that you like, nothing that you ought to have. Perhaps a set of scales. Maybe storage boxes to refrigerate left overs, and save them from getting snatched into your hands and posted to your stomach so quickly that they hardly touch the side of your mouth. You might choose readymade and measured meals in your cupboard, to help you adjust to calorie counted portions and avoid unwelcome supermarkets for a while, until you feel more confident. Have healthier, easy to grab foods available to you so you have something to satisfy urges and cravings.

You'll have heard this before, no doubt, but our point is this – be *honest*, be *assertive,* be *clear* with yourself and those sharing your environments, and take control, not make excuses. Environments influence habits- make yours work to support your journey of controlling your *physical* self through your *mental* mechanisms and practical actions.

Of course the home is largely under your control. What about those other challenging environments we find ourselves in, other peoples' `gardens' such as the work canteen, the restaurant with friends, the cinema, or the motorway service station, for example? Choices can be tempting. And sometimes environments trigger old behaviours! It's easy to think of what you `always do', or can `never do' - `I always have popcorn when I go to the cinema', `I always have a bacon sandwich at work', `I can never get time for exercising when I'm working all over the place.' If these sorts of beliefs and thoughts crop up when you change environment, then do two things. One is consider how you might change old patterns from the inside out, and revisit your beliefs, as in The Hare and The Tortoise.

The second thing is to acknowledge that, from the outside in, preparation and planning is key. Pack up some food to take on your journey, buy a small bag of healthier popcorn to take to the cinema, or only eat a third of the box if you used to eat a whole box. Consider before going to the restaurant what courses you might indulge in. These decisions and actions become the physical tools of an effective weight management programme. You will also need to rely on yourself – Mary knew what she wanted in her garden, so made whatever efforts she needed to in order to get them. You need to do the same. Remember your planned outcome, and in challenging environments, use mental mechanisms to make changes. You might order starters without main course, share a pudding – anything that is conducive to changing your habits in a way that will *honestly* support the direction of your weight loss.

`What *specific* tools do you think I might need?' Mary pondered with the gardener. `And it needs to be something for all seasons, because weather changes, nights get longer, plants grow at faster or shorter rates, flower at different times.'

`Well, Mary. I suppose that depends again on your own unique garden. You will feed more at some times than others, because more energy is given to growth at different times. You will need the right clothes to protect yourself, and the right machines and hand held gadgets for pruning and tidying.'

Specific tools for weight loss can be snack packs, reminders of our goals, whatever works. Gardening is of course a very active pursuit, and you, like Mary, might need the right tools to integrate a little activity in your life. If you're away a lot, find an exercise habit that you can do anywhere – take exercise bands, take trainers, take a swimming costume – easy and light to pack. Buy weights, have a machine at home, get some great dance music to move to. Think carefully about this, and only buy if you are at the stage of `I will lose and manage weight forever', rather than `I ought, I should lose weight.' Because we have a hunch that there are millions of ab fabbers, exercise balls and running machines sadly rotting under beds or in garages! The *tool* is exactly that – not something to do the job *for* you, but something to help you do the job when you are absolutely sure that you want the job done. And start small –a pair of secateurs and shears is not too much of an investment for the small gardener, just like the exercise band and the trainers, music or swimming costume. The trick is to give yourself choice and manage yourself in any surroundings, keeping your weed killer and your insect repellent in your bag, and your sense of contentment and control in your mind.

If you have the will and the right tools, preparing your environment will pay huge dividends in changing your behaviour. For holidays, or meals out, plan ahead- imagine the environment before you get there and rehearse how you will manage. When it comes to food, you know, nothing is of itself deadly (other than poison); it's just how much of it you have and how you balance it out in your life that counts towards your goals. If you insist on feeling deprived by eating less, then you are doomed. If you begin to savour everything, only eat when you're hungry and stop when you're full – if you balance your calorie seesaw in your particular garden, so that neither side is too loaded – you can do anything.

Now and then, things shout a little loudly. When we enter a supermarket, or a restaurant, or pass a fish and chip shop, an Italian restaurant, an Indian take away, for example, our senses are alerted and trigger hunger or desire. We become conditioned, by associating certain smells, music, or images to something we know and trust, or to a memory of something that has excited or satisfied in the past. Those cunning restaurateurs and other food vendors use this knowledge to get us to buy and then eat THEIR product...how rude is that?

Well guess what? You can be just as cunning, and with a bit of planning, defeat those clever dicks. YOU can grow what you want, plant your own crops, choose what fragrances you want to stimulate you, choose your own images, and excite yourselves with well formed outcomes always in your mind. You can create your own internal secret garden. This is the knack of taking yourself inside when all else is shouting at you, finding a place of inner peace where you can arrange everything to your own satisfaction, and breathe easy as you do so.

But that's another story – and you'll find it on our MP3 where Graham will help you go inside at any time you like to remember to have control over where you are in your own environment.

To finish up, let's just go back to Mary Quite Contrary. She worked hard at her garden, planted her pretty maids all in a row, and then arranged her cockle shells and silver bells just where she wanted them.

And then invited her gardener mentor round to have a look.

'Well, Mary', he said, smiling with pleasure. 'Look at all those changes you've made, you've fined everything down and got all your plants to the peak of health. And now you've got a lovely little path carved out for yourself.' He smiled at the cockle shells. 'And those are most unusual, though they blend very well. What about the bells, Mary, what inspired those?'

Mary grinned.

'Well, they're my little reward to myself. Every time I got one flower bed nearer to where I wanted to be, I bought myself a silver bell to give myself a pat

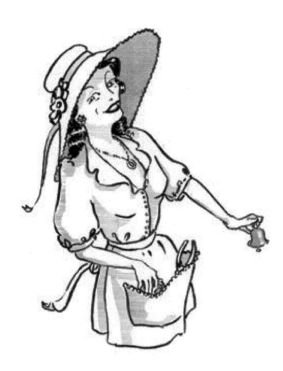

on the back, and hung it in the garden where I could see it to encourage me. And now I have a whole line of lovely twinkly bells that look pretty all around me and make this place really my own.'

My three most challenging environments are:
1.

2.

3.

Now consider all the tools and resources that you have within you and around you to take into those environments to make the desired changes. For example, if the kitchen leftovers are the most challenging, then start to buy less food, or cook less food, or put leftovers immediately into the freezer or the bin. Become conscious of how much food you are actually making. If restaurants are tricky, pre plan with the menu in mind, use the mental resource of imagining how you will feel half an hour after eating, and so on. For each environment, rehearse and write down how you can best look after yourself in that environment – because you *are* worth it. And equally, as you make changes within yourself, you may find, that some environments become less attractive. Write down your thoughts and plans below or in your notebook.

Environment One

WHAT I WANT IS:

WHAT/WHO I HAVE TO HELP ME ARE:

WHAT I MIGHT SAY IS:

WHAT I WILL DO DIFFERENTLY IS:

Environment Two

WHAT I WANT IS:

WHAT I HAVE TO HELP ME ARE:

WHAT I MIGHT SAY IS:

WHAT I WILL DO DIFFERENTLY IS:

ENVIRONMENT THREE

WHAT I WANT IS

WHAT/WHO I HAVE TO HELP ME ARE:

WHAT I MIGHT SAY IS:

WHAT I WILL DO DIFFERENTLY IS:

REMEMBER, MAKING SUSTAINABLE CHANGES
IS EASY IF YOU HAVE A CLEAR PICTURE OF
WHERE YOU ARE GOING. USE ALL OF THE
RESOURCES THAT YOU NEED, AND REHEARSE
EVERYTHING THAT YOU WILL DO AND SAY TO
GET THERE.

The End - and the Beginning

Well, we hope you have enjoyed this book and that it leaves you with much food for thought ☺, and with the confidence to be just the person who you know yourself to be. Our aim is for you to synthesize your mind and body in a way that is comfortable and true to yourself, or at least to be on the first step of that journey. We're here in this particular life but once, so it can be really helpful to make yourself the best fit possible, to enjoy being here.

Remember you can download the MP3, either of the book or of the trances, if you feel that will help.

Whatever your choices, don't wait to manage weight – stop talking, start doing. This is your life, your body, your mind, and it's time to create your own weight management programme with a truly fairy tale ending. Enjoy.

Who's Broken My Scales is supported by a set of MP3 light trance inductions which allow you to make changes easily and quickly while in a very relaxed state. Visit www.e-junkie.com/WhoBrokeMyScales to download.
There is also an e-book version available on lulu.com and soon to be available on amazon.co.uk and amazon.com

Dr Jan Russell Dexter is an accredited Coach (AC, ILM), writer and a Senior Fellow in Coaching at the University of Lincoln, teaching to MSc level. She is also a Practitioner, Master Practitioner and Trainer in Neuro Linguistic Programming.

Jayne Hildreth has a Graduate Diploma in Counselling, and an MSc (Distinction) in Personal and Corporate Coaching. She works as a freelance coach, counsellor and trainer. Jayne lectures in counselling and coaching to Bsc for Hull University..

Dr Graham Dexter is an accredited Coach (AC), Master of Education, and Senior Fellow in Coaching at the University of Lincoln, teaching coaching to MSc level. He is an NLP Master Practitioner, and a world expert on Birmingham Roller Pigeons.

All three offer personal coaching and coaching workshops.

When you have enjoyed this book, you might be interested in:

Dexter, J, et al (2011) *An Introduction to Coaching.* London: Sage
Dexter, J and Dexter, G (2009) *Blank Minds and Sticky Moments in Counselling* London: Sage

Other books by the authors include:
Dexter, G (1997) *Winners with Spinners (the art of high quality pigeon cultivation.*
Russell, J (2009) *Keeping Abreast* (fiction)
Russell, J. (2009) *Rough Diamonds* (fiction)

Contact Janice@healthandlifetransitions.com for more info regarding publication, coaching and workshops